for
Diabetes
Relief

YOGA
for
Diabetes
Relief

Bharat Thakur

Copyright © 2007, Bharat Thakur

ISBN 81-8328-060-9

All rights reserved. No part of this book may be reproduced, stored in a retrieval system or transmitted in any form or by any means — electronic, mechanical, photocopying, recording or otherwise — without the prior permission of the publishers.

While every precaution has been taken in the preparation of this book, the publisher and the author assume no responsibility for errors or omissions. Neither is any liability assumed for damage, if any, resulting from the use of information contained herein.

Published by

Wisdom Tree
4779/23 Ansari Road
Darya Ganj, New Delhi-110002
Ph: 23247966/67/68

Printed at

Print Perfect
New Delhi-110064

Contents

1	Yoga and Health	1
2	Understanding Diabetes	3
3	Managing Diabetes through Yoga	9
4	Dietary Regulations	13
5	Diabetes Management Programme	17
	Beginner's Programme	22
	Shatkarma	23
	Pranayama	32
	Bandha	38
	Asana	46
	Mudra	90
	Relaxation	96
	Meditation	100
	Advanced Programme	104

1

Yoga and Health

"The only healthy man is a Buddha."

Health, as we know it to be, does not merely mean the absence of disease. Health is a positively vibrant state of being that the individual experiences through his efforts. According to Ayurveda, a man is healthy when he is able to forget his body, or in other words, when the body is in such a state that it is not a source of ache, pain or illness, and the individual feels light, free and 'uncaged' by the body.

Physical well-being is absolutely necessary, but it is only a beginning. In yoga, it is said that the physical body is one of the sheaths of our being. We have the following five sheaths or *koshas*:

- *Annamaya kosha* refers to the gross physical body
- *Manomaya kosha* refers to the mental body (thoughts)
- *Pranamaya kosha* refers to the subtle energy body
- *Vignanamaya kosha* refers to the psychic body
- *Anandamaya kosha* refers to the transcendental, blissful body.

One can be healthy only if all these levels of being are pure. Hence, we can conclude that our health is also determined by what we think and how we feel about our self and our life. The process of being healthy is, in other words, an ongoing process of growth.

How does all this relate to diabetes and diabetics?

As of today, modern medicine says that there is no positive system of cure for diabetes. It says *that diabetes is an incurable disease that can only be managed.* Medicines, we know, can only control the symptoms of diabetes, but the disease is not really affected by this mode of treatment, and may even develop in severity.

In contrast, yoga therapy for diabetes begins on a positive note — that the disease can be managed successfully and perhaps, even eliminated. Yoga works successfully in the management of diabetes because it taps the body's innate regenerative ability. Rather than approaching the disease from the outside, yoga approaches it from within, relying on re-balancing of the nervous system, re-stimulation of the endocrine glands and pancreas, and improvement of the physical organism and its energy flow. All these together with meditation set the stage for the patient's recovery and a deeper understanding of himself, which is the key to eliminating psychosomatic diseases.

Practicing yoga causes an enhanced state of relaxation, improving stamina and immunity towards disease. An overall improvement of physical health and mental well-being is seen.

2

Understanding Diabetes

Diabetes (diabetes mellitus) is a disease caused by the presence of abnormally high levels of blood glucose in the body. Glucose is the fuel for the cells of the body. When we eat food, the carbohydrates present in what we eat get converted into glucose inside the body. This glucose is then absorbed as a fuel by the cells of the body. The absorption is facilitated only by insulin, which is a hormone secreted by the beta cells of our pancreas. When glucose enters the body, it triggers the release of insulin from the pancreas, thus 'pushing' glucose into the cells of the body and also into the liver and fat cells, where it is stored. Hence, without insulin any amount of glucose in the body is useless, as it cannot get absorbed by the cells.

The balance is maintained in the body by a hormone called glucagon which is secreted by the alpha cells in the pancreas. It works contrary to insulin and is released when the body is starved or undergoes strenuous exercise. Glucagon triggers the release of stored glucose in the body in order to feed the cells.

Diabetes occurs due to a deficiency in insulin production or insulin action, causing blood glucose levels to rise dangerously and leading to serious complications and, maybe even, premature death.

There are primarily two types of diabetes and these are described below:

Type 1 Diabetes (Juvenile Onset Diabetes)

Type 1 diabetes accounts for 5 to 10 per cent of all cases of diabetes and is an auto-immune disorder in which the body mistakes the beta cells of the pancreas (which are responsible for producing insulin) to be invaders and attacks them. Slowly as more and more beta cells disappear, the body becomes incapable of producing insulin (or produces it in very small amounts), causing diabetes to develop. Patients suffering from this type of diabetes are afflicted in their childhood or youth. Patients are forced to use insulin injections or pumps. A controlled diet and regular exercise are recommended for these patients.

Type 2 Diabetes (Adult Onset Diabetes)

Type 2 diabetes accounts for 90-95 per cent of all diabetes cases. Here insulin is produced by the body but in very small amounts, which is insufficient or the insulin produced is not utilised by the cells properly, leading to insulin resistance. As the need for insulin increases, the pancreas needs to overwork and may gradually lose the ability to produce insulin.

Type 2 diabetes is usually associated with people over 40 years of age (although these days, it is seen even in people who are 25 years of age). Patients of Type 2 diabetes are often overweight, lack physical exercise and have a family history of diabetes or of gestational diabetes.

Gestational Diabetes

Gestational diabetes is a form of glucose intolerance diagnosed in some women during pregnancy. It is more common among obese women and in women with a family history of diabetes. During pregnancy, treatment is required to normalise the maternal blood glucose levels so as to prevent complications in the infant. Nearly 70 per cent of the women who have had gestational diabetes tend to develop Type 2 diabetes at some point of their lives.

Other types of diabetes result from specific genetic conditions (as maturity-onset diabetes in youth), surgery, drugs, malnutrition, infections and other illnesses. They account for 1 to 5 per cent of all diabetes cases.

Symptoms of Diabetes

The following are the symptoms of diabetes:
- Unusual thirst
- Frequent urination, especially at night
- Excessive hunger
- Abnormal weight loss
- Blurred vision

- Irritability
- Increased fatigue
- Slow healing of wounds
- Itching around the genitals

Complications due to Diabetes

Not only is diabetes a degenerative disease, the patient is also at a higher risk of developing the following:

- heart disease and stroke
- nephropathy or kidney failure
- high blood pressure
- neuropathy or nerve damage, especially in the legs (leading to amputation)
- retinopathy or damage to the eyes, that can lead to blindness
- dental disease
- sexual dysfunction
- pregnancy complications

Aim of Treatment

The prime aim of treatment or management of diabetes is to maintain blood glucose, blood pressure and cholesterol levels as near as possible to normal. When this happens, either the medication is reduced or stopped completely.

Pre-diabetes

Pre-diabetes is a condition where the blood glucose levels are higher than normal but not high enough to be diagnosed as diabetes. For those who are not diagnosed with diabetes, there remains the risk of pre-diabetes. If you are diabetic, chances are high that some of your close relatives have pre-diabetes. Patients who develop Type 2 diabetes almost always have pre-diabetes.

Adults who are overweight and 45 years of age or older are prone to develop pre-diabetes. If you have any of the other risk factors for diabetes, such as high blood pressure, low HDL cholesterol and high triglycerides, or a family history of diabetes, the chances are more of your suffering from pre-diabetes.

What must an individual with pre-diabetes do?

Studies show that if you manage your blood glucose levels when you have pre-diabetes, you can delay or prevent the onset of Type 2 diabetes. It is also possible to return your blood glucose levels to the normal range through changes in lifestyle.

The treatment recommended for people with pre-diabetes is moderate weight loss (5-10 per cent of total body weight) through diet and basic physical exercises, such as walking or yoga, for a minimum of 30 minutes a day, five times a week.

Hypoglycaemia

Hypoglycaemia, or low blood sugar is a condition that most people have experienced at some stage of their life. Hypoglycaemia can happen to the diabetic due to excessive intake of insulin, causing blood sugar levels to fall abnormally or it can be precipitated due to intake of an excessively sugary diet. This will result in the blood sugar rising alarmingly, causing insulin to be over-secreted as a reaction. Immediately after experiencing a high, the person feels a low due to lack of glucose in the blood. The brain is starved and one experiences tiredness, irritability and depression. Other symptoms include headache, poor concentration and forgetfulness. A person suffering from hypoglycaemia experiences disturbing fluctuations between high and low energy states.

Patients are advised to carry a small piece of pure glucose (like a candy) with them. This is for an emergency situation. When the blood sugar level drops too low, then the patient may even enter into coma that can prove fatal. Hence, it is better to immediately have some glucose. If the condition does not improve, immediately rush to a hospital or a doctor.

The causes of hypoglycaemia include chronic stress, lack of exercise and consumption of an excessively sugar diet. To overcome hypoglycaemia, dietary and lifestyle changes are recommended.

3

Managing Diabetes through Yoga

As we have seen, diabetes is a psychosomatic disease, i.e. a disease that affects the mind-body matrix. These factors are both genetic and environmental, hence we list diabetes as a lifestyle disease. While modern medicine can take care of the symptoms of diabetes, it requires the efforts of the patient himself to develop the awareness to eliminate the root cause out of his system. In other words, the patient is the most important factor in his diabetes management.

Know that all diabetics are advised to do exercise every day. This is an absolutely vital cog in the management of diabetes, along with medication and diet. However, there is something still missing — and that missing element in diabetes management is relaxation.

Relaxation is extremely important for your body, mind and soul. No system in the world has understood relaxation as deeply as yoga. Relaxation does not mean watching TV, listening to music or simply sitting idle. These are merely sensory distractions, whereas relaxation is a deep unwinding and release of physical, mental and emotional intensions. The mind is all-pervasive and in yoga we say that the body and mind are aspects of the same phenomenon. Hence, stress caused to one aspect will adversely affect the other.

The most important step in relaxation is to learn how to counter stress in life. The practice of *yogasana*, *pranayama* and meditation will help you to deal positively with stress.

Firstly, stress causes an increase in the activities of the sympathetic nervous system and the adrenal gland. This results in the release of more glucose into the blood. Next, the hormonal secretions of the pancreas are controlled by the autonomic nervous system. Mental or emotional tension can disturb the normal functioning of the autonomic nervous system and of the endocrine glands, thus inhibiting the secretion of insulin. Hence we find that prolonged stress can lead an individual to develop diabetes.

Why is doing *asanas* better than any exercise?

Your doctor must have told you all about the need to exercise as part of your diabetes management programme. The minimum recommended exercise is 30 minutes daily, five times a week. This could include brisk walking, jogging, yoga, weight training, dancing, aerobics, tennis, and so on. Exercise is emphasised because studies show that exercise improves the absorption of glucose, besides enhancing the overall health and well-being of an individual.

Any exercise or fitness regimen must comprise cardio-vascular endurance, flexibility and strength training. Yoga is the only discipline that provides all these three fitness elements.

Yogasana, while giving the practitioner the physical benefits of exercise, works on a deeper level. *Asanas* are postures that open the body so that energy can flow easily, toning the body, while stressing and massaging the internal organs so that there is increased blood supply to these areas and their functioning improves.

Practicing *asanas* regularly impacts the nervous system, endocrine system and metabolism better than exercise. This, we know, is vital in diabetes management.

Shankhaprakshalana

The *hatha yoga* practice of *shankaprakshalana* is known to greatly reduce the levels of blood sugar in the body, almost as soon as the patient begins its practice. *Shankhaprakshalana* is the process of systematic cleansing of the alimentary tract which runs from the mouth to the anus. The complete exercise is done only once a season or twice a year. It is absolutely necessary that this be done under the guidance of a qualified yoga teacher.

Laghoo shankhaprakshalana is the shorter version of the practice. It is seen to have the desired effect of lowering the blood sugar levels just as *shankhaprakshalana* does. The practice involves drinking a number of glasses of warm, saline water and practicing a set of five *asanas*, that open the sphincters in the alimentary canal, allowing the water to pass through and out of the anus. The practitioner will automatically pass stool at first and by the end, only clear water will pass out through the anus. The alimentary tract, including the stomach and intestines, is thus cleansed of any residual waste matter.

Now the practitioner must rest. This is the only time that the digestive system (including the pancreas and the liver) gets to rest, as the intestines are completely empty.

It is imperative that the blood sugar levels are checked, because they tend to fall dramatically when *laghoo shankhaprakshalana* is practiced. Hence, insulin dosage must be modified appropriately, or in many cases, even stopped during the days the patient practices *laghoo shankhaprakshalana*.

Meditation and Diabetes Management

The modern man portrays an image of deep insecurities and the hectic pace of life leaves him/her feeling exhausted and estranged.

Meditation helps us untangle and resolve the underlying tensions that affect the personality. Often the root cause of diabetes and other psychosomatic diseases lies in the underlying tensions. Meditation helps to calm, relax and reconnect to our spiritual being, thereby leading to bliss in daily life and a higher level of awareness. Finally it is found that yoga and medication work together, making the patient more receptive to treatment.

4

Dietary Regulations

Since diabetes is a disease caused by imbalance in the metabolism, the diet of the patient becomes a key factor in its management. Every diabetic patient should consult a dietician for specific dietary advice that takes his lifestyle and cultural preferences into account.

If you are overweight, losing weight slowly will help you control your diabetes. Do not try to lose weight in a hurry by crash dieting; instead try to lose weight gradually.

Creating a Meal Plan

For a diabetic patient, when he eats is as important as what he eats. The meal plan should be scheduled around your insulin injections or medication, if you are taking them. This is because insulin has peak times when it works the most. Meals and snacks should be planned around such timings to ensure that you get the energy from food when insulin is at its highest. Secondly, once the insulin is injected, it works no matter what the blood glucose level in the body is. Hence, if there is too little glucose in the blood when insulin is at its highest, you could experience hypoglycaemia (low blood glucose). Hence is important to abide strictly to the meal timings as far as possible.

Foods

The building blocks of all the foods that we eat are:

- *Carbohydrates*: Carbohydrates are the body's main source of fuel. Our digestive system turns carbohydrates into glucose which feeds all the cells of the body. Carbohydrates influence blood glucose levels more than any food. Hence it is important to keep a track of the amount of carbohydrates contained in your meal.
- *Proteins*: The main job of proteins is to build and repair the tissues in your body. Proteins can also be used as a fuel but it takes double the time for proteins to be converted into glucose.
- *Fats*: Fats are the reserve fuel in the body, or in other words, concentrated energy. They also help in the absorption of certain vitamins. However, they have double the calories as carbohydrates and proteins. Eating too much of fats can make you overweight and clog your blood vessels, leading to complications of the heart.
- *Vitamins and minerals:* These are needed for your body to work well and are mostly found in food which is rich in carbohydrates and proteins. The best way to get all the different vitamins is to eat different kinds of foods, especially fruits and vegetables.

- The American Diabetic Association recommends a diet in which 60 to 70 per cent of calories come from carbohydrates, 20 to 30 per cent from proteins and 10 to 20 per cent from fats.

Dietary Guidelines

- A *high fibre* diet is highly recommended. This includes whole grains, beans and vegetables. Studies show that adopting a high fibre diet reduces insulin dosage in many cases.
- It is beneficial to eat more *complex carbohydrates*, such as wheat, buckwheat, oatmeal, corn and wholegrain (unrefined) rice. Complex carbohydrates are broken down slowly, so that the body has energy for a longer time and the blood glucose level does not shoot up immediately.
- Avoid eating simple sugar, such as white sugar, honey, glucose, chocolate and other sweets, including the traditional Indian sweets.
- Maintain a low-fat diet because high fat diets impair the carbohydrate metabolism and increase the chances of falling prey to heart disease, which most diabetics are prone to.
- Salt intake should be low.
- Alcohol intake should not be too high (consult your doctor).

Sugar and Sugar Substitutes

A common diabetic myth is that people suffering from diabetes can never eat sugar. This is because sugar raises the blood glucose level rapidly. However, recent research has shown that all carbohydrates affect your blood glucose levels in the same way.

You can savour sweet foods occasionally as part of a balanced diet. You must plan this and ensure that you have enough insulin in the body to handle the carbohydrates in the sweets and the consequent increase in blood glucose levels. Another option is the use of sugar substitutes, that are used with tea or coffee. Calorie-free sugar substitutes do not contain carbohydrates, so your blood glucose levels will not rise.

5

Diabetes Management Programme

Normally when a diabetic patient wants to begin yoga therapy, he will need to start with relaxation practices, followed by *asana*, *pranayama*, *shatkarmas* (cleaning techniques) and meditation. It is necessary to maintain this holistic approach so as to reach a state of relaxation, bring down the blood glucose levels and develop the strength of body and mind needed to eliminate the root cause of the disease.

This programme is for patients who suffer from diabetes, without the manifestation of other complications like heart disease or blood pressure. It is important that each patient consults a qualified yoga therapist and his doctor, before beginning the practice, in order to chalk out an individual programme for himself/herself.

Two programmes are outlined here and these include a programme for beginners, irrespective of whether you have done yoga before or not; the second should be commenced only after you feel comfortable in doing the exercises advised in the first programme.

Commencement of the Programme

> *"Atha yoganushasanam."*
>
> — *Patanjali Yoga Sutra*:1

Patanjali says, '*Atha yoganushasanam*', which means, 'now the discipline of yoga'. By 'now', Patanjali means that before one enters yoga, one has to learn to be aware of the fact that one cannot perform yogic practices without being totally focused on the present moment.

Yoga is practiced in a relaxed atmosphere, so before starting on it, bring yourself to a relaxed state. Sit comfortably with your back straight, and count from one to 10. Compose yourself, tell yourself that for the next one hour (or for whatever time you practice), you will completely focus on your yoga, and not think about your work or home or family and other commitments. Gift yourself this time!

Essentials of Yogic Practice

Place

One should try to practice yoga in an open space as far as possible. It is advisable to practice yoga in a nice clean room with natural lighting in the morning, or gentle lighting for the evening.

Timing

The best time to practice yoga is on an empty stomach at sunrise, when the weather is pleasant and before you get busy with your daily routine. Sunset time is also good for yoga, as it is a calm and serene time of the day that helps you to unwind peacefully. The sunset time is extremely good for meditation.

Duration

The duration of the yoga session which should range between 40 minutes to one-and-a-half hours. This should suffice to complete the programme.

Breathing

Breathing is a very important aspect of yoga. A simple rule to follow is to inhale when you bend backwards and exhale while bending forward. Whenever you hold a posture, breathe normally, except when indicated otherwise.

Pace

The pace of yogic postures (except for *surya namaskar*) should be very slow and should be practiced in steps. To move from one basic position into another within the same *asana* is an *asana* in itself.

Clothes

One should either wear loose-fitting or skin-tight clothes that allow plenty of freedom of movement in all directions.

Equipment

There is no specific equipment required for the practice of yoga.

However, one can use ropes, bricks, round pillows, elastic belts, and, of course, the yoga mat.

Fragrance

Natural fragrance is the best as flowers, plants and trees, soil, etc., all have their own aroma. If one does yoga in a room, one should always burn an incense stick or an aromatic candle. This makes you feel more relaxed and focused.

Music

Maintaining a posture and fixing the mind beyond is the basic technique of doing an *asana* as nothing can be better than the natural surroundings — the music of chirping birds, the rustle of leaves or jumping of squirrels on branches. However, you can also listen to devotional music, or else, if you appreciate Indian classical music, songs based on *ragas* are the best option.

Regularity

One has to be very regular with yogic practices as muscles and joints take a lot of time to become flexible, though stiffness and rigidity return very easily. Practicing for four days and missing one day means going back to square one, hence such is the importance of regularity.

Medical problems

People with specific medical problems should consult their doctor before they practice certain *asanas*. Do not assume that you will be alright. Apart from hypoglycaemia, high blood pressure and heart disease, conditions such as cervical spondylitis restrict you from doing certain *asanas* and *pranayama*. Normally if you suffer from high blood pressure, avoid holding your breath in the *pranayama* exercises and avoid undertaking inverted postures.

Order of yogic practices

One should always practice *pranayama* and then move on to *bandhas*, *kriyas* and lastly, *asanas*. *Pranayama* needs a pattern of relaxed breathing. If one practices *pranayama* after the *asanas*, then the breathing pattern becomes faster, which is not good for *pranayama sadhana* (practice). *Bandhas* are followed by *pranayama* because certain *bandhas* are done along with *pranayama*. The rest of the *bandhas* can be done later. The *mudras* given for diabetes management involve the whole body, so it is better to practice the *asana*, relax, and then do the *mudras*, as the body is more open and flexible. *Mudras* are followed by relaxation and subsequently by meditation. The programmes have been chalked out in the right order to be maintained by the practitioner.

Programme 1 or Beginner's Programme

Shatkarma	*Laghoo shankaprakshalana*
	Kunjal kriya
	Jala neti
Pranayama	*Bhramari pranayama*
	Bhastrika pranayama
Bandha	*Mool bandha*
	Uddiyaan bandha
	Agnisaar kriya
Asana	*Pawanmuktasana* series
	Tadasana
	Tiryaka tadasana
	Kati chakrasana
	Trikonasana
	Surya namaskaar
	Meru wakrasana
	Baithak merudandasana
	Marjariasana
	Ushtrasana
	Janusirsasana
	Bhujangasana
	Paschimottanasana
	Pawanmuktasana (*ekpad* and *poorna*)
	Merudandasana
Mudra	*Sharnaghat mudra*
	Yoga mudra
Relaxation	*Shavasana*
Meditation	*Ajapa japa*

SHATKARMA

Shatkarmas are purification practices. In the yoga tradition, *hatha yoga* comprised the *shatkarmas*, which consisted of six groups of exercises performed to achieve physical and mental purification and balance. They are also used to achieve balance between the three *doshas* (humours) in the body — *kapha,* mucus; *pitta*, bile and *vata,* wind.

The six groups of *shatkarmas* are *neti, dhauti, nauli, basti, kapalbhati* and *trathak*. For the purpose of diabetes management we shall practice *neti* and *dhauti*.

Neti is the process of cleansing and purifying the nasal passages and includes the practice of *jala neti* and *sutra neti*.

Dhauti is a series of cleansing techniques and are divided into three categories. We use the *antar dhauti* or internal cleansing technique, which includes *shankaprakshalana* or *laghoo shankhaprakshalana, agnisar kriya, kunjal kriya* and *vatsara dhauti*.

A word of caution

The *shatkarmas* are highly specific and powerful practices which should be learnt correctly under the guidance of a qualified yoga teacher.

Practice notes

Laghoo shankaprakshalana can be practiced after about two weeks to a month from the start of the programme. Actually twice a week is ideal and after a month, once a week is sufficient (depending on the patient's condition). *Laghoo shankhaprakshalana* is followed by the practice of *kunjal kriya* and *jala neti*. *Jala neti* however, is practiced daily. The blood sugar level must be monitored as it tends to drop dramatically when these practices are started.

Poorna shankhaprakshalana, an extended form of the practice, is performed once a season and under the guidance of a qualified yoga teacher. Patients are recommended to consult a yoga teacher before attempting this exercise.

LAGHOO SHANKHAPRAKSHALANA (intestinal wash)

Laghoo shankhaprakshalana, is one of the most important yogic practices that helps to bring down the blood glucose levels.

It should be done on an empty stomach early in the morning. No tea, or even fruit, must be consumed before starting the practice.

- Prepare three litres of lukewarm water and a teaspoon of salt for each litre. The water must taste mildly salty. For patients suffering from high blood pressure, do not mix salt in the water.
- Drink two glasses of the prepared water rapidly.
- Perform the following five *asanas* eight times each: *tadasana, tiryaka tadasana, kati chakrasana, tiryaka bhujangasana, and udarakarshanasana* (described in the advanced programme section). Perform these *asanas* at a steady pace in quick succession, without taking a break.
- Drink two more glasses of water and repeat the five *asanas* eight times each.
- Repeat the process for a third and last time.
- Go to the toilet but do not strain yourself even if there is no bowel movement. If there is no motion immediately, it will come later on. Wait patiently for this to happen. Usually, after the practice, there is full bowel discharge including discharge

of plenty of urine.
- Finally *kunjal kriya* and *jala neti* can be done.

Rest

- On completion of the practice, rest for half an hour. Keep yourself warm, but try not to sleep. You can lie down or sit down.

Food

After resting, eat *khichdi* — a special preparation made with rice, pulses (*mung dal*) or lentils, and cooked in *ghee* (clarified butter) as it provides protection to the inner walls of the stomach and intestine, while the body provides a new inner layer. (Often the inner layer of the stomach gets stripped along with the residual waste present in the stomach.) Even if you are not hungry, you must eat this meal. Later in the day, try to not to consume refined or non-vegetarian food and alcohol, especially the first few times you attempt the practice.

Benefits

- Encourages normal functioning of the intestines.
- Brings down blood glucose levels dramatically.

KUNJAL KRIYA (regurgitative cleansing)

This Kriya is done on an empty stomach in the early morning hours and following the practice of *laghoo shankhaprakshalana*.

- Prepare about two litres of lukewarm water by adding two teaspoonfuls of salt. For patients suffering from high blood pressure, do not mix salt in water.
- Stand near a sink or outside, in the garden.
- Drink at least five glasses of the prepared water at one stretch. Ensure that you gulp down the water and do not sip it slowly.
- Stand with the legs apart and the back bent forward.
- Place the index, middle and ring fingers in the mouth (ensure that the hands are clean and the nails cut) and rub the back part of the tongue. This stimulates the vomiting process. Water will start coming out of the mouth.
- Wait till all the water comes out. If the vomiting stops, again rub the back of the tongue with the fingers. Ensure that all the water comes out.
- Once all the water comes out, then relax for a while and do deep breathing.

Benefits

- Tones the abdominal organs, removing indigestion, acidity and gas.

- Removes excess mucus, thus helping to cure cold, cough, bronchitis and asthma.
- Helps release pent-up emotions and blocks, or heaviness in the heart caused by inner and outer conflicts.

Contraindications

- This should be avoided by people suffering from hernia, high blood pressure, heart disease, stroke, acute peptic ulcer or diabetics with eye problems.

JALA NETI (nasal cleansing with water)

A special *neti lota or neti* pot with one end ending in a nozzle in required. The should fit comfortably in the nostril.

- Prepare lukewarm water by adding one teaspoonful of salt per half litre. Fill a little water in the *neti* pot.
- Stand with the legs apart and bend slightly forward.
- Tilt the head forward to one side and breathe deeply.
- Place the end of the nozzle in the nostril that is facing upwards and let the water flow slowly into the nostril. Do not force it.
- Slowly the water will enter the nostril and flow out through the other nostril.
- When the water has flowed out, straighten the head and blow out through the nostril to gently to remove the excess mucus.
- Repeat with the other nostril.
- On completing this step, dry the nostrils by performing *kapalbathi kriya* with one nostril closed and then the other for three minutes.
- Perform *kapalbhati kriya* with both the nostrils open. Take in a deep breath and exhale forcefully through the nostrils, pulling in the stomach each time you exhale. Exhalation is active while inhalation is passive. Continue to exhale till you are out of breath. Take in a deep breath and begin to exhale once again. Repeat three times.

Benefits

- Removes mucus and pollution from the nasal passage and the sinuses.
- Prevents respiratory tract diseases such as asthma, pneumonia, bronchitis and pulmonary tuberculosis.
- Relieves disorders of the ears, eyes and throat, including myopia, allergic rhinitis, hay fever and tonsilitis.
- Alleviates muscular tension in the face and imparts a youthful appearance.
- Removes anxiety, anger, depression and drowsiness while improving the activities of the brain and overall health.
- Perform the *kapalbhati kriya.*

Contraindications

- This exercise should be avoided by people who suffer from chronic bleeding of the nose.

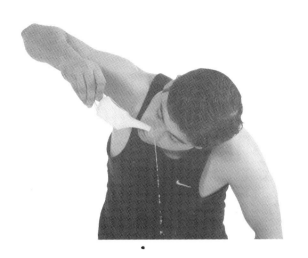
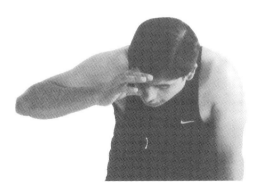

PRANAYAMA

Prana means 'breath' and *ayam* means 'control'. *Pranayama* is the art of wishful awareness of the entire breathing system; it is a form of meditation. Practice of *pranayama* strengthens the lungs, calms the nerves, restores, equalises and gradually balances the flow of vital energy to the brain, the other organs and the glands. It also reduces stress levels, which is so important in the management of diabetes.

Note

Pranayama must be practiced for at least 15 minutes daily. Begin by performing for five minutes and gradually increase the duration of your practice. The best time to practice *pranayama* is early morning.

Pranayama is usually practiced by sitting in *padmasana* or *vajrasana*, both of which are meditative poses. You can also sit on a chair with you back straight, if sitting on the floor is difficult.

- *Padmasana* (lotus pose): Bend one leg, and place your ankle on the opposite thigh, close to the groin.
- Bend the other leg and place the ankle on the thigh of your bent leg, close to your groin.
- Place your hands on your knees (see photos on *pranayama*).
- *Vajrasana*: Kneel down.
- Bring your feet together and interlock your big toes.
- Slowly sit down by bringing your buttocks on to the insides of your feet and place your hands on your knees.

BHRAMRI PRANAYAMA

- Sit in *padamasana* or *vajrasana*. You can also sit on a chair with you back straight, if sitting on the floor is difficult.
- Close your eyes and take a few deep breaths.
- Place your thumbs in the ears to keep them closed. You should not be able to hear any outside sound. Your fingers are placed on top of your head.
- Inhale deeply, counting till five while inhaling.
- Hold your breath by pressing your chin down to your jugular notch and perform the *jalandhar bandha* (described in detail under **Bandhas**).
- Raise your chin up so that the head is straight and create a humming sound, like that of a bumble bee, from your throat, with your voice moving upwards towards the head. Allow the whole vibration to spread all over the head.
- Practice all the three parts in a rhythmical pattern. Try and see how many counts of inhalation you can do so that you can continue the same for some time without getting tired. Do not over-hold the breath, else your next round won't be the same as the previous one.

Benefits

- It sends a vibratory massage to the brain cells so that all the blood vessels and nerves which are constricted (vasoconstricted) get transformed into a state of vaso-dilatation. The brain is brought to rest because of which some anti-stress hormones get secreted.

- This is a form of meditation, which helps to develop the art of focussing, consequently developing memory power and higher mental faculties.
- It relaxes the vocal chords and improves the quality of sound.

Contraindication

- People with severe throat problems like throat concer should avoid this.

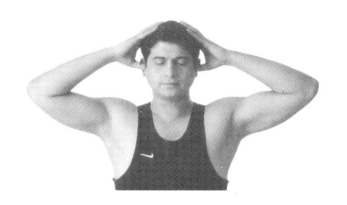

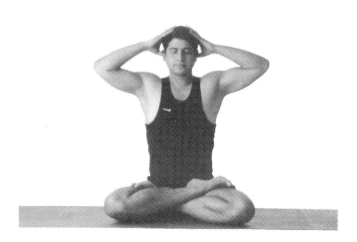

BHASTRIKA PRANAYAMA (bellows' breath)

- Sit in *padamasana* or *vajrasana*. You can also sit on a chair with you back straight, if sitting on the floor is difficult.
- Bend the arms at the elbows, keeping them close to the waist and close your hands into fists.
- Inhale deeply and raise both the fists up, a bit higher than the head, keeping the elbows close to the body.
- Exhale forcefully through the mouth (cheeks puffed out) as you pull the arms down, taking the elbows behind the waist as shown.
- Repeat this 20 times. Inhalation is deep and slow, whereas exhalation should be rapid, with smooth movements.

Benefits

- This is the only *pranayama* that removes all ailments related to the three *doshas*: *vata*, *pitta* and *kapha*.
- It is very good for one's mental and physical health.
- Cures depression, tiredness, insomnia, phobia and anxiety.
- Gives one a feeling of calm and peace.
- Awakens the *chakras* and the *kundalini*, unleashing one's inherent power.

Caution

- Do not move while practicing *bhastrika*.
- Breathe through the lungs only, without inflating your belly.

Contraindications

- Do not hold your breath if you have high blood pressure, heart disease or neurological problems. Take care to breathe very slowly.

BANDHA

In yoga, *bandhas* are the neuromuscular locks that regulate and increase endocrine (glandular) secretions in the body, including the pancreas that secretes insulin. The endocrine glands are ductless glands which are essentially porous in nature. By performing *bandhas*, the glands are pressed and activated, thus enhancing the secretion of hormones.

Together with other yogic practices, they help improve the hormonal balance in the body, the metabolism, and most importantly, reduce the stress levels. The hormonal levels in our body determine our moods and frame of mind, so by performing the *bandhas* one can feel more relaxed and happy. Reduction in stress levels automatically affects the blood glucose levels positively, thus enhancing insulin secretion.

There are three *bandhas* in yogic practice: *jalandhar, mool* and *uddiyaan bandhas*.

- *Jalandhar bandha* regulates the secretions of the thyroid and parathyroid glands. Thyroxin secreted by the thyroid gland helps to regualte the metabolism and body temperature. The secretion of the parathyroid gland is crucial to the proper functioning of the immune system of the body.
- *Mool bandha* regulates the secretions of the sex glands, as well as the adrenal and pancreatic glands. This helps to improve the vitality and energy levels of the individual.

- *Uddiyaan bandha* regualtes the secretions of the adrenal and pancreatic glands, including insulin. This has a beneficial effect on the blood glucose level in the body.

The three *bandhas* must be practiced every day, since they directly affect the homeostasis (internal hormonal environment) of the body.

A note of caution

- Each *bandha* should be practiced only three times in a day.

MOOL BANDHA (root lock/perineum contraction)

- Sit in *padmasana* or *sukhasana* with eyes closed on a chair with your back straight and legs kept apart, if sitting on the floor is difficult.
- Exhale deeply through your mouth and hold your breath.
- Close your anal space and raise the lower abdominal organs and muscles to hold as long as possible.
- Release slowly the lower abdominal organs.
- Inhale and relax your body, bringing your breathing back to normal.
- Practice three times.

Benefits

- Strengthens the lower abdominal muscles, the excretory system and the glands in the abdominal area.
- Helps women suffering from several gynaecological problems.
- Improves problems like asthma, bronchitis and prostrate.

Contraindications

- Should not be practiced by pregnant women.
- Persons with heart disease or high blood pressure should avoid this practice.

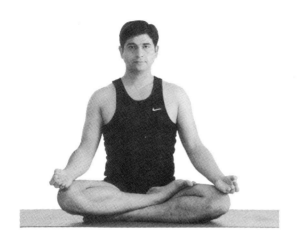

UDDIYAAN BANDHA

- Stand with your legs apart and inhale.
- Exhale completely, and bend forward, placing your palms on your thighs, just above the knees. (The palms are turned inwards with the thumbs pointing upwards.)
- Pull in your stomach to create a hollow space.
- Hold as long as comfortable, with the breath held inside.
- Release the contraction in the stomach, stand up and breathe in. Exhale that breath.
- Again breathe in.
- Exhale.
- Repeat the entire practice.
- Practice only three times.

Benefits

- Helps to change the pressure inside the abdomen. Research indicates that there is a pressure change of -20 to -80 mm of Hg during the practice of *udyaan bandha*, allowing the release of more gastric juices which help in the digestive process.

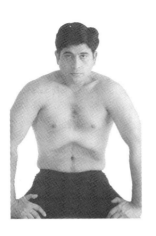

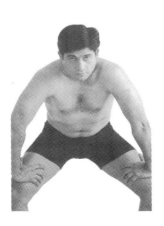

AGNISAR KRIYA

- Stand with your legs apart and inhale.
- Exhale completely through the mouth, and bend forward, placing your palms on your thighs, just above the knees. (The palms are turned inwards with the thumbs pointing upward.)
- Holding your breath, pull your abdominal muscles inwards to create a hollow space.
- Continue to hold your breath and push your abdominal muscles out. Create a rhythmic movement — pulling the stomach inside and pushing it out.
- Repeat this cycle 10 to 70 times.
- Slowly build up your stamina and increase the number of rounds you can perform.

Benefits

- Improves the peristaltic movement of the stomach and helps to digest food better.
- Stimulates the functioning of the adrenal and pancreatic glands.
- Helps to remove constipation.
- Strengthens the abdominal muscles and removes fat from the abdominal area.

Contraindications

- Consult your doctor if you have undergone stomach surgery.

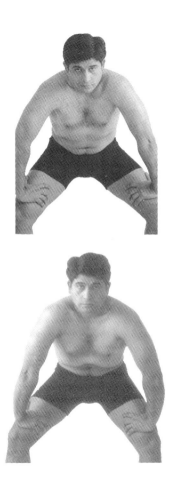

ASANA

Yogic *asanas* not only tone and exercise the body but stretch the internal organs so that there is increase in blood supply to these areas and their functioning improves. The *asanas* selected work on the endocrine system, particularly the glands. The benefits of practicing *asanas* have been dealt with in the previous chapter. *Asanas* work on both the outer framework of the body such as the muscles, joints and skeletal structure, and the inner system of the body. For example, a side stretch — *trikonasana*, may appear to be beneficial in toning the sides only, but it also has a positive effect on the internal organs and endocrine glands in that area. By massaging and stretching the glands, the secretions of these glands is regulated.

Yogis understood the importance of hormones and hormonal balance long before modern medical science could even detect their presence. Hence a large amount of the practices in yoga directly manipulate and regulate hormonal secretions.

Definition of asana

In the *Yogasutras* of Patanjali, *asana* is referred as '*sthiraha sukham asana*', meaning 'stability and well-being in an *asana*'. This refers to the fact that the goal of practicing *asana* is to be able to sit in one of the meditative postures for a long period of time, comfortably and unmoving. This is a pre-requisite for the practitioner to experience meditaion.

How to practice asanas?

Patanjali says, "*Prayatna saithilyam anantha samap prathibyan*," which means one should effortlessly try to perform a posture by fixing the mind beyond. By 'beyond' he means that one should not think of mundane issues in life while practicing the *asanas*. One should be aware of things like one's breath, music, or movement from one position to the other or the target muscle that is stretched to the maximum.

Practice note

The sequence of *asanas* mentioned in the following pages is important. The programme begins with the *pawanmuktasana* series for loosening up the joints in the body.

Pawanmuktasana Series

NECK ROTATION

- Sit comfortably with your back straight and lower your head down.
- Gently rotate your neck in a complete circle.
- Repeat this procedure five times.
- Practice five times in the reverse direction.

Benefits

- Relieves tension in the neck and shoulders.
- Removes stress from deskwork.
- Helps to prevent cervical spondylitis.

Contraindications

- People with cervical spondylitis should perform this very gently, after consulting their doctor.

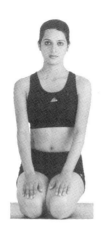
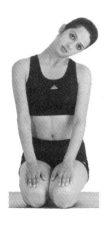
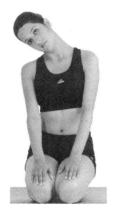

SHOULDER SOCKET ROTATION

- Sit comfortably with your back straight.
- Fold your elbows and place your fingertips on your shoulders.
- Rotate your shoulders.
- Repeat five times.
- Reverse the direction and repeat five times.

Benefits

- Relieves strain of driving and deskwork.
- Helps relieve cervical spondylitis and frozen shoulder.
- Tones the muscles of the chest and shoulders.

Contraindications

- People suffering from frozen shoulder should check with their doctor before attempting this exercise.

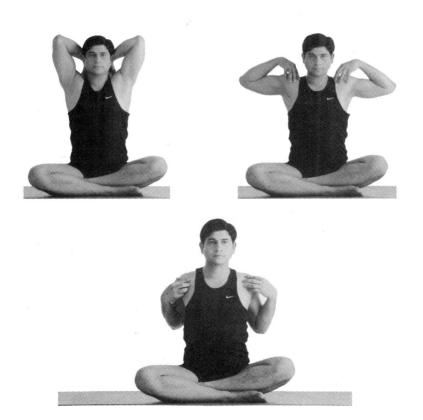

WRIST AND ANKLE FLAP

- Sit comfortably with your back straight and legs stretched out.
- Stretch your arms out and move your wrists so that your palms are turned inward and fingers point downward.
- Simultaneously, bring your toes inward and hold for a few seconds.
- Move your wrists so that your palms are turned outward, and fingers point upward.
- Simultaneously, push your toes outwards. Hold the posture for a few seconds.
- Repeat this cycle 10 times.

Benefits

- Improves circulation in the forearms and legs.
- Loosens the wrist and ankle joints.
- Helps relieve stress.

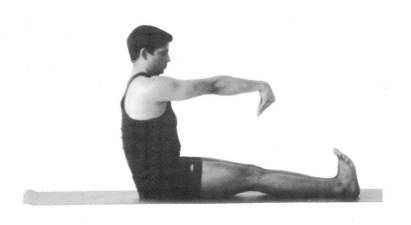

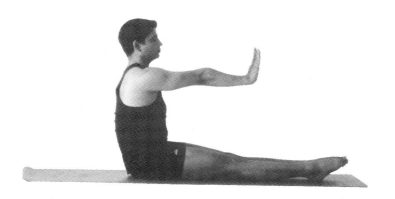

KNEE PRESS

- Sit comfortably with your back straight and legs stretched out in front.
- Bend your right leg at the knee and pull it in with both hands, pessing against your trunk. Raise your upper body and touch your chin to your knee. Hold for a few seconds.
- Repeat with your left leg.
- Pull both the legs to your chest and keep them pressed tightly. Then release your legs.
- Repeat five times.

Benefits

- Frees the knee joint.
- Helps in opening up the groin area.
- Assists in relieving the knee pain.

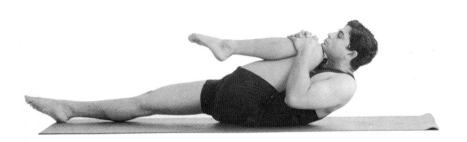

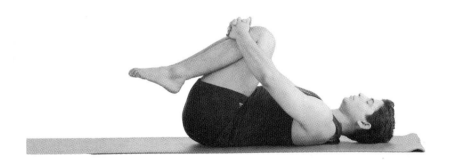

TADASANA

- Stand with s gap of one foot between your legs and raise your hands over the head.
- Raise your heels up and stretch your whole body up as high as possible.
- Join your hands and hold the posture for 30 seconds to a minute, breathing normally throughout the practice.
- Slowly bring your hands back and exhale.
- Place your heels on the floor and hands by the side of the thighs.

Benefits

- Helps to remove stiffness from the spine, tiredness from the upper part of the body and strengthens the ankles and the smaller joints of the foot.
- Improves the strength of the calf muscles.

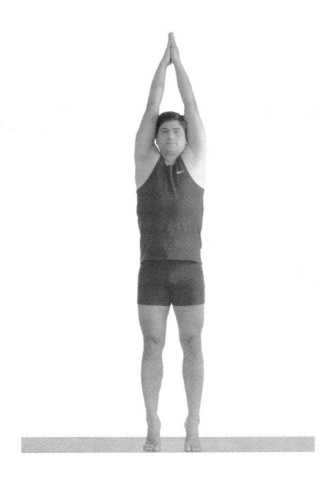

TIRYAKA TADASANA

- Stand with your legs apart and raise your hands above the head.
- Grip the right wrist with the left hand.
- Exhale, keeping the head and eyes straight ahead.
- Bend to the left from the waist, for 10 to 30 seconds, breathing normally.
- Inhale and come up.
- Repeat on the opposite side.

Benefits

- Stretches sides of the trunk, exerting a mild, beneficial pressure on the pancreas. (Together with other yogic practices, this pressure may help stimulate the pancreas in the production of insulin in Type 2 diabetic patients whose insulin production is just below the threshold level. Further the pancreatic and adrenal glands, and the liver, get massaged and toned).
- Strengthens the back muscles.
- Improves flexibility of the spine.

Contraindications

- Those with frozen shoulder should not practice this *asana*.
- Persons with severe back problems should consult a yoga therapist or their doctor.

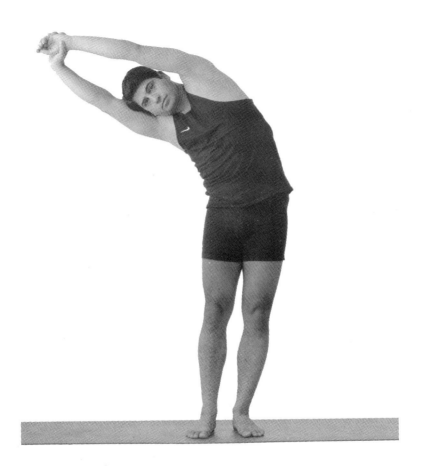

KATI CHAKRASANA

- Stand straight with the neck relaxed.
- Bend your elbows.
- Place one palm on the opposite shoulder and place the other hand behind your back.
- Turn your back and head and look over your shoulder on which the hand rests.
- Hold the posture for 10 to 30 seconds.
- Repeat by interchanging the position of your hands and twist to the other direction.

Benefits

- Stretches the side of the trunk, exerting a mild pressure on the pancreas.
- Proves beneficial in correcting postural problems.
- Relieves stiffness and pain the back.

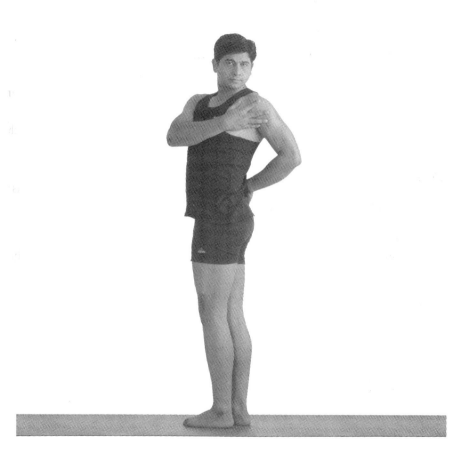

TRIKONASANA

- Stand with the legs apart and the left arm placed under the armpit.
- Bend sideways, exhaling slowly till your right hand goes below the right knee.
- Hold the posture for 10 to 30 seconds and breathe normally.
- Repeat it on the other side.

Benefits

- Actively stretches the waist area and exerts a mild pressure on the pancreas.
- Tones the sides of the body.
- Helps to remove fat from the outer sides of the thighs.

Contraindications

- Those with high blood pressure and vertigo should not practice this *asana*.
- Those with severe back problems should avoid *asana*.

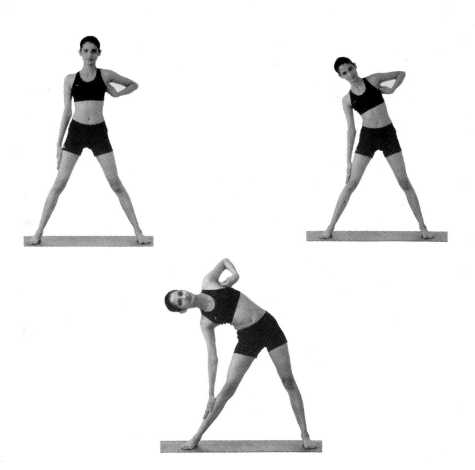

SURYA NAMASKAR

Surya namaskar or sun-salutation is a combination of 12 *asanas* used as a warming up exercise before practicing and performing the other *asanas*. It affects practically every muscle of the body and its regular practice ensures good health, flexibility and strength.

Surya namaskar works on more than just the physical dimension. It requires you to co-ordinate your breathing with each movement and each posture has an accompanying chant that is recited mentally. Awareness is always maintained on the muscles that are stretched or on one's breath. For the advanced practitioner, awareness is maintained on the *chakras*.

Begin with a practice of five to 10 rounds, before reaching 20 to 30 rounds. Yogis are known to do as many as 108 rounds at one time.

- Stand straight with palms folded in front of your chest and feet kept together.
- Breathe normally, chanting the *mantra*, "Om mitraya namaha."
- Inhale and stretch your hands over your head, locking the shoulders and the ears together and stretch backwards while chanting the *mantra*, "Om ravaye namaha."
- Exhale and bend your body forward till your fingers, palms or hands touch the floor by the side of your feet.
- Try and touch your knees with your forehead and relax, while chanting the *mantra*, "Om suryaya namaha."
- Inhale and take your left leg back and place both your palms on the floor by the side of your right leg.

- Arch your back and avoid touching the left knee on the floor, chanting the *mantra*, "*Om bhanave namaha.*"
- Exhale and bring the right leg back and make a straight line from the head to the toe with the body weight balanced on the toes and palms. Chant the *mantra*, "*Om khagaya namaha.*"
- Hold your breath and place your knees on the floor.
- Bend your elbows, pressing your chest and forehead on the floor. In this position your toes, knees, chest and forehead touch the ground, while you chant the *mantra*, "*Om pushnaya namaha.*"
- Inhale and stretch your upper body upwards.
- Straighten your elbows and arch the back to look up, while chanting the *mantra* "*Om hiranya garbhaya namaha*".
- Exhale and raise your hips upward as high as possible, tucking the chin inwards towards the chest and looking at the navel. With your heels pressed on the floor, chant the *mantra*, "*Om marichaya namaha.*"
- Inhale and bring your left leg forward arching the back, as in the fourth position, chanting the *mantra*, "*Om adityaya namaha.*"
- Exhale and bring both the legs forward and touch your toes as in the third position, chanting the *mantra*, "*Om savitre namaha.*"
- Inhale and stretch your hands over your head backwards as in the second position, chanting the *mantra*, "*Om arkaya namaha.*"
- Exhale and come back to the first position, chanting the *mantra*, "*Om bhaskaraya namaha.*"

Benefits

- *Surya namaskar* improves the flexibility of the whole body.
- Proves effective in weight loss, provided one starts with 10 rounds and goes up to 51 to 108 rounds within two or three months.
- Stimulates the functioning of the endocrine system.
- Opens the *granthis* (the physical blockages of the body) and makes the body look younger, vibrant and lustrous.
- Improves the auto-immune system of the body.
- Balances all the vital plexus of the body from the *mooladhar* (the root plexus) to the *brahamarandra* (the crown plexus).

Caution

- Start slowly and gradually increase your stamina with the number of rounds you perform.

Contraindications

- Overweight or obese persons should start slowly. Do not get discouraged by the movement involved. Initially it seems difficult, but within a few sessions the rhythm of the movement will become ingrained in you.
- Persons with high blood pressure or heart disease, should not hold their breath in the positions.

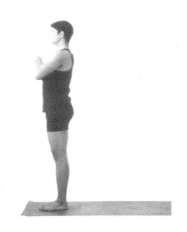
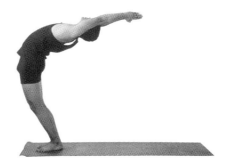
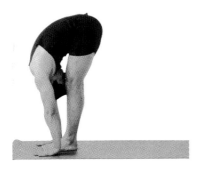
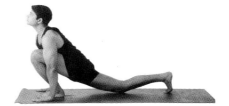

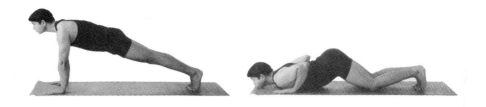
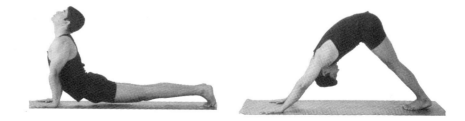

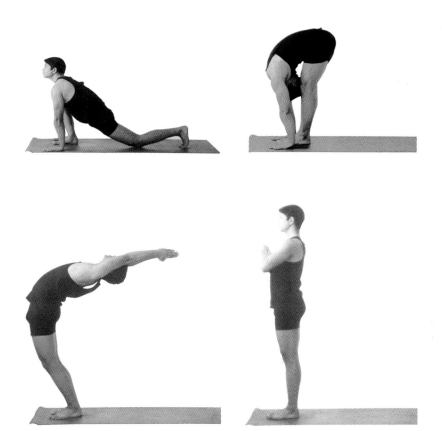

MERU VAKRASANA (sitting spinal twist)

Spinal twists are considered important in the programme for a diabetic, as they apply a beneficial pressure on the internal organs of the body, especially the pancreas.

- Sit with the legs outstretched, back straight.
- Bend the right knee.
- Bring the left hand to the outer side of the right leg, twisting the trunk.
- Place the left hand on the floor near the right ankle.
- Place the right hand behind the back on the floor for support.
- Turn the back and look over the right shoulder.

Benefits

- Stretches the spine, loosens the vertebrae and tones the spinal nerves.
- Exerts a mild pressure on the pancreas.
- Relieves sciatica, lumbago and neck pain.

Contraindication

- People with severe back problems, ulcer and hernia should avoid this posture.

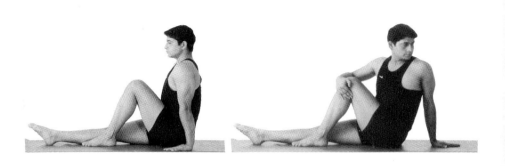

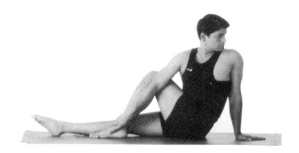

BAITHAK MERUDANDASANA

- Sit with your back held straight and both arms placed behind as shown.
- Bend one leg, and place the foot on the kneecap of the other leg.
- Gently twist the spine, taking the knee towards the floor on the opposite side.
- Hold the position for 10 to 30 seconds, breathing normally.
- Repeat on the other side.

Benefits

- Loosens up the spinal column and helps relieve lower backache.

Contraindications

- People suffering from severe back spasms, such as scoliosis, should avoid this *asana*.

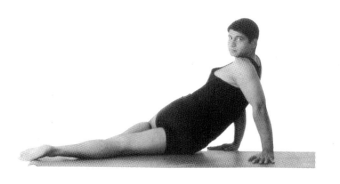

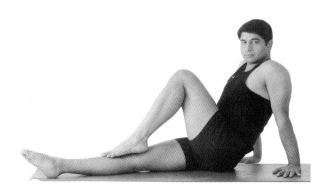

MARJARIASANA (cat stretch)

- Place your palms and knees on the ground.
- Inhale and look upwards, arching your back and head upwards.
- Exhale and curve your back inwards to look at your navel.
- Repeat this movement about 10 times.

Benefits

- Improves the flexibility and strength of the back.
- Removes the postural defects of the back, like a rounded back or lordosis (a back in which the lower waist is ahead of the midline of the body).

Caution

- Perform this *asana* very gently and slowly and avoid jerks.

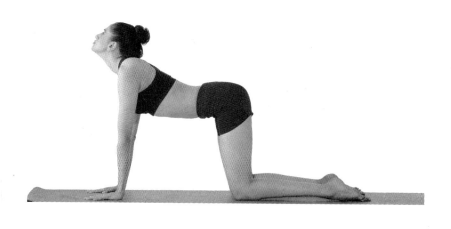
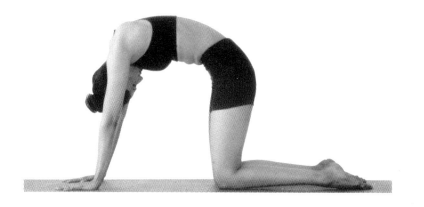

The following set of *asanas* alternately stretch the back forward and backward, maintaining the spine flexible and strong while, toning the abdominal area and the internal organs.

USTRASANA (camel pose)

- Kneel down with the knees held a little apart and feet stretched out.
- Lean back, catch hold of right heel with the right hand and then the left heel with the left hand.
- Push the abdomen forward, drop the head back and arch backwards as far as you can.
- Hold as long as comfortable, breathing normally.
- Slowly release one hand, then the other and return to the start position.

Benefits

- Stretches the abdominal area, helping to remove excess weight.
- Strengthens the lower back and neck muscles.

Contraindications

- People with a severe backache should avoid this *asana*.
- Those suffering from cervical spondylitis should be careful while stretching the neck backwards.

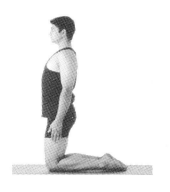

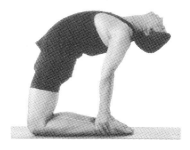

JANUSIRSASANA

- Sit with your back straight and legs stretched out.
- Bend one leg and place it so that the heel touches the groin area.
- Inhale and raise your arms up, straight.
- Exhale, bend forward to grasp the foot or ankle (or shin) of the outstretched leg, and bring the forehead down to touch the knee.
- Hold for 10 to 30 seconds.
- Repeat with the other leg.

Benefits

- Stretches the hamstring muscles of the thighs.
- Helps to remove the excess weight in this area.
- Increases the flexibility of the back and hip joints.

Contraindication

- Those with lower back problems should avoid this *asana*.

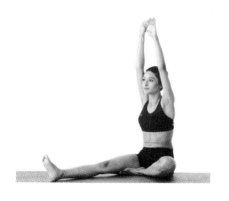

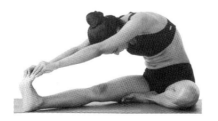

PASCHIMOTTANASANA

- Sit on the floor with your legs stretched out in front, feet kept together and hands resting on the sides.
- Inhale and raise the arms upward, keeping the back as straight as possible.
- Slowly exhale and bend forward from the hips, trying to hold your toes with your fingers.
- Hold this position for a few seconds.
- Continue exhaling and further lower the back, trying to touch your forehead to the knees by resting your elbows on the ground.
- Breathe normally and hold the posture for 10 to 30 seconds.

Benefits

- Stretches the hamstring muscles of the thighs.
- Helps to remove excess weight in this area.
- Increases the flexibility of the back and hip joints.

Contraindication

- Those with lower back problems should avoid this *asana*.

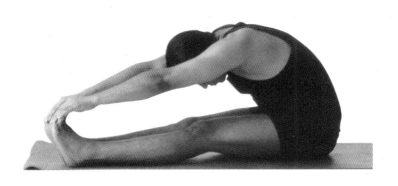

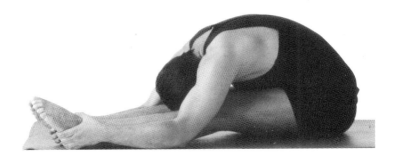

BHUJANGASANA (cobra pose)

- Lie on your stomach with the chin touching the ground, legs straightened out and toes tucked in. Place your arms next to the shoulders, elbows close to your chest.
- Raise your chest and arch your back, keeping your elbows bent and navel touching the ground. Look towards the sky and continue to hold this position for a few seconds.
- Raise your thighs off the ground and hold for a few seconds, while breathing normally. Practice when the back is flexible and strong.

Benefits

- Helps to remove stiffness from the front part of the body including the chest, shoulders and neck.
- Stretches the abdominal muscles and helps to remove flab from the abdomen.
- Cures urino-genital problems in males and gynaecological problems in women.
- Removes lower back pain by strengthening the back muscles.

Contraindication

- People suffering from hernia, hydrocil, spinal injury and those who have undergone stomach surgery should avoid this *asana*.

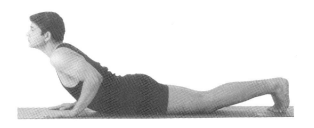

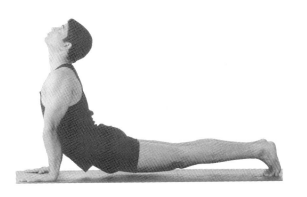

EKPAD PAWANMUKTASANA

- Lie flat on the back, hands kept by the side of your thighs.
- Interlock your fingers, bend your right knee, place your hands over your knee and slowly exhale while pulling your knee towards your chest.
- Raise your upper body and bring your chin over your knees.
- Hold still for 30 seconds to a minute, breathing normally.
- Relax your grip, straighten your leg and come back to the lying-down position. Repeat on the other side.

Benefits

- Removes lower backache or stiffness from the lumbar region.
- Stretches the hamstring and the hips, removing extra fat from these areas.
- Improves flexibility of the hip and knee joints.
- Rids you of gas problems.

Contraindication

- People suffering from cervical spondylosis should not raise their body up and bring it over the chin. They should keep their head on the floor.

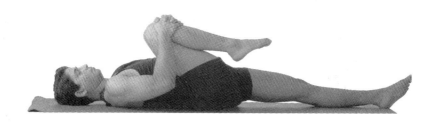

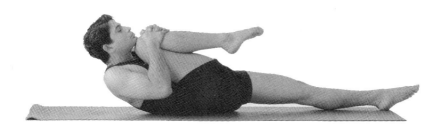

85

POORNA PAWANMUKTASANA

- Lie flat on your back with your arms by your side.
- Inhale, clasp both the knees with your hands and bring them close to your chest.
- Pull your upper body and bring your chin over your knees.
- Hold the posture for 30 seconds to a minute and breathe normally.
- Relax your grip, straighten your legs and return to the lying-down position.

Benefits

- Reduces stiffness from the lower back.
- Removes fat from the hips.
- Fights pain in the knee joint.
- Helps to remove unwanted gas from the body

Contraindication

- People suffering from cervical spondylosis should not raise their body up and bring it over the chin. They should keep their head on the floor.

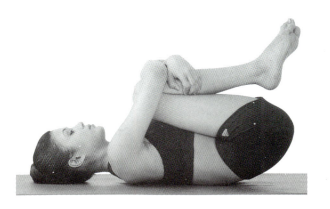

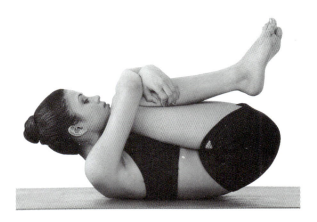

MERUDANDASANA (spinal twist)

- Lie down on your back, hands outstretched.
- Place your right foot on your left knee.
- Exhale and twist your back, taking your right knee across the body to the left and try to touch it to the floor, looking to the right.
- Hold the position for 10 to 30 seconds, breathing normally.
- Repeat on the other side.

Benefits

- Helps in removing stiffness and pain from the upper and mid back.
- Makes the back more flexible.
- Gives a massage to the internal organs of the stomach.
- Stretches the trapeze muscles (muscles above the collar bone) removing stiffness from the neck.
- Stretches the sciatic nerve, controlling the sciatica pain.

Contraindication

- People suffering from severe sciatica should consult the doctor before practicing this *asana*.

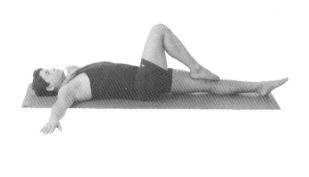

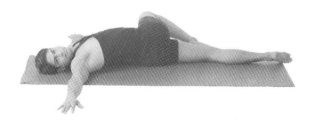

MUDRAS

In yoga, *mudras* are a combination of physical movements, attitudes and gestures that focus on changing the homeostasis (internal hormonal environment) of the body. They improve the functioning of the endocrine system and the glands in the body. Practicing of *mudras* helps to de-stress and induce a relaxed state in the person's mood.

The practice of *mudras* is highly subtle and requires the practitioner to be already proficient in *asana*, *pranayama*, and *bandha*. *Mudras* have a deep effect on the working of the body and mind. Many of the yogic *mudras* must be learnt from the guru by the *shishya* (disciple). However, the *mudras* given in the following pages are simple and can be practiced for relaxation.

Yogis researched with the human body and discovered that certain gestures or *mudras*, positively influenced the functioning of internal organs, galnds and systems. For example, in *Hriday Mudra*, by placing the tip of the thumb to the tips of the middle and ring fingers, and the tip of the index finger to the base of the thumb, the functioning of the heart improves. Medical research is now beginning to prove the beneficial effects of *mudras*.

The beauty is that they not only affect the physical organism, but have a more subtler effect on the body-mind matrix, or in other words, the psychosomatic dimension of the individual. *Mudras* influence the moods of the practitioner. Hence it is possible to minimise stress, and other afflictions such as mood swings and tempers, and so on. This brings the practitioner into a balanced state of existence, which is conducive not just to health but also to relaxation and meditation.

Caution

Certian *mudras* may produce results that the individual is not equipped to handle. Hence *mudras* are introduced later, once the individual is grounded in the practice of yoga. However, the *mudras* mentioned in the following pages are relaxing in nature, and can easily be practiced.

SHARNAGHAT MUDRA

- Sit in *vajrasana*.
- Inhale and raise your hands above your head.
- Exhale slowly while bending your body forward from the waist till your forehead touches the floor.
- Let your buttocks touch your heels.
- Relax in this posture for 30 seconds to a minute, before breathing normally.
- Slowly come up and while coming up, inhale.

Benefits

- Removes stiffness from the back.
- Improves blood flow to the head, particularly to the brain cells, energising and relaxing the upper body.
- Removes pimples and dark circles under the eyes and makes the face look fresh and healthy.
- Helps to check problems like headache or sinus.

Contraindications

- People suffering from lower backaches or high blood pressure should avoid doing the *sharnaghat mudra*.

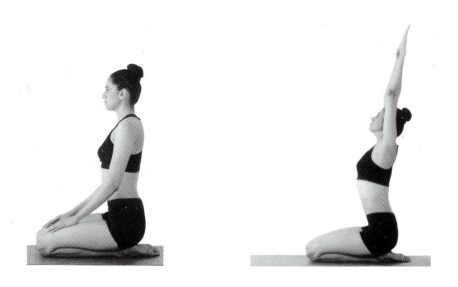
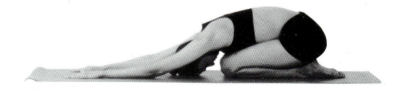

YOGAMUDRASANA (psychic union pose)

- Sit in *padmasana* or, in *ardha padmasana*.
- Close your eyes, breathe deeply and relax.
- Take your hands behind your back and hold one wrist with the other hand.
- Exhale slowly and bend yourself downwards, taking your forehead towards the floor. Relax and breathe normally in this posture for as long as is comfortable.
- Inhale deeply and return to the starting posture. Repeat by interchanging the position of the legs (place the other leg on top in *padmasana*). Practice the posture two to three times.

Benefits

- Massages the abdomen and helps to tackle ailments of the organs in this area, notably indigestion and constipation.
- Massages the internal organs, including the pancreas.
- Stretches the spine, thus toning the spinal nerves between the spinal discs.

Contraindications

- To be avoided by people suffering from severe eye, heart or back problems.
- Not to be practiced by people in the early post-operative or post-delivery stage.

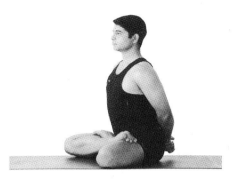

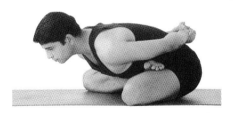

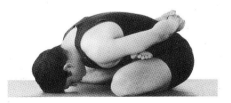

RELAXATION

As seen earlier, relaxation is an integral part of diabetes management. Relaxation does not mean 'doing nothing', for even when we are not doing something, the mind is still racing, pondering over all kinds of thoughts. Relaxation is a deep unwinding of physical, mental and emotional tensions. We may be working or driving or doing something, but it is possible to remain relaxed.

Relaxation must be a part of everything we do so that we may thoroughly enjoy our life. Practicing yoga helps us to relax and become stronger, thereby preventing us from getting tense or stressed easily. We develop the strength to remain unaffected by what would have previously seemed highly stressful situations. Practicing these simple relaxation techniques slows down the breathing and produces a calm state of mind that continues throughout the day, even after completing the yoga practice. This is as vital for each and every person as it is for the diabetic.

Yoga says that stress is an unnatural state of existence and that relaxation is the natural state of existence for an individual. Yoga calls this *anandamaya chitta* or blissful state. The present state that we find ourselves in is called *vikshipta chitta* or diseased state. More so in our modern times, with a hectic pace of life, man is unable to slow down his mind or remain focused on any one thing for a longer duration. He spends his day roaming from one distraction to another, just as the average person keeps flipping TV channels. It is important that man finds time for leisure, at least one hour daily. This helps the individual to unwind and let go. Otherwise the stress keeps building up for years together and ultimately mainfests in disease of one kind or the other. Leisure and relaxation become all the more important given the nature of our nuclear families, and our own loneliness.

SHAVASANA (corpse pose)

Shavasana is deeply relaxing and is practiced at the end of the *asana* session for the body and mind to rest and rejuvenate. It is recommended even to insomniacs and others who cannot relax.

- Lie flat on the back with your legs slightly apart.
- Let your hands lie loosely by your sides, with your palms facing upward.
- Close your eyes and relax.
- Practise deep abdominal breathing. As you breathe in, the stomach rises and as you breathe out, the stomach falls down.
- Begin a countdown of your breaths, starting at 11 and count down till you reach 0 (11 deep breaths). After a few weeks, increase your countdown from 27 to 0.

Benefits

- Relaxes the entire body and mind, removing physical and mental tiredness.
- Helps one fall asleep.
- Develops awareness of the body and mind.

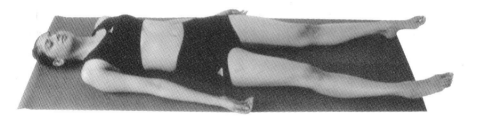

MEDITATION

Meditation has a beneficial effect on every level of the individual (*refer* to Chapter 3). The practices detailed here are those that specifically help the diabetic. Once you have mastered these, you will find that meditation becomes an integral part of your life, just as sleeping or eating. Be diligent with your practice even though it may seem tedious or boring at first. The mind will slowly begin to balance between introversion and extroversion, while ceasing to hanker for excitement in the outside world.

Once this happens, you will be richly rewarded with a relaxed frame of mind, happiness, improved overall health and a higher state of awareness.

Meditation can be practiced either immediately after finishing the programme or at night before going to sleep. It is up to the practitioner, although meditation before sleeping proves relaxing and helps you unwind and enjoy a restful sleep.

AJAPA JAPA

Japa means chanting or remembering of a *mantra*. This could be a *mantra* given by a guru or if you do not have a *mantra*, then the *mantra* of breath, *'so-ham'*, is used. In *japa*, the *mantra* is consciously repeated within the mind to create permanent awareness. As the practice becomes more and more grounded in the person, the conscious chanting of the *mantra* is slowly replaced by an unconscious chanting or by *ajapa japa*.

- Sit in a meditative posture (in *padmasana*, *vajrasana* or *sukhasana*) or else sit on a chair with your back straight.
- Place the back of your palms on your thighs. Join the tips of your thumbs to the tips of your index fingers in *dhyaan mudra*.
- Keep the eyes closed.
- Breathe deeply for a few minutes, being completely aware of each and every breath — inhalation and exhalation. All breathing should be done through the nostrils.
- As you breathe in, your chest and rib cage expand, while the stomach is drawn in slightly. As you exhale, the chest drops down and the stomach returns to its normal position.
- Co-ordinate your breath with the chanting of the *mantra*. As you breathe in, simultaneously start chanting *'so'*. While you do this, bring awareness to your navel at the start of the breath, and slowly imagine it moving upwards from the navel to the throat. Hold your breath for a second before exhaling.

- As you exhale, simultaneously chant *'ham'*. When doing this, bring your awareness to your throat, and slowly start imagining it move downwards from the throat to the navel. On reaching the end of exhalation, re-start inhalation. In this manner you will be chanting, *'so-ham'*, as you practice one complete breath.
- Continue this practice for five minutes.

As you become more proficient and enjoy the practice, increase the duration to 10 to 20 minutes. Then bring this slow breathing and chanting into your everyday life while travelling, cooking, relaxing or so on. By and by, you will become a much more relaxed person.

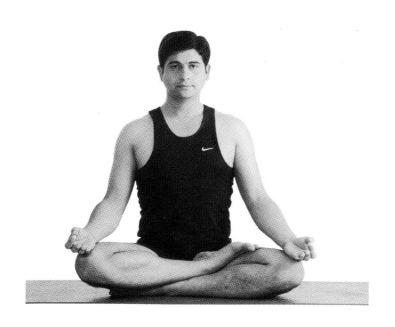

Programme 2 or Advanced Programme

Shatkarma	*Jala neti*
	Kunjal kriya
	Laghoo shankaprakshalana
Pranayama	*Bhramari pranayama*
	Anulom-vilom pranayama
	Bhastrika pranayama
Bandha	*Udyaan bandha*
	Mool bandha
	Mahabandha
	Agnisaar kriya
Asana	*Pawanmuktasana series*
	Tadasana
	Tiryaka taasana
	Kati chakrasana
	Trikonasana
	Surya namaskaar
	Baithak merudandasana
	Ardha matsyendrasana
	Gomukhasana
	Marjariasana
	Ushtrasana
	Janusirsasana
	Bhujangasana

	Tiryaka bhujangasana
	Dhanurasana
	Paschimottanasana
	Naukasana
	Pawanmuktasana (ekpad and *poorna)*
	Merudandasana
Mudra	*Sharnaghat mudra*
	Vipareet karni mudra
	Matsyasana
Relaxation	*Shavasana*
Meditation	*Ajapa japa*
Yoga nidra	

The advanced course programme begins just the same way as the beginners' programme. The advanced yogic practices that are not included in first programme are found here.

ANULOM-VILOM PRANAYAMA

- Sit in *padamasana* or *vajrasana*. You can also sit on a chair with your back straight, if sitting on the floor is difficult.
- Close your eyes and take a few deep breaths.
- Bend the index finger and middle finger of your right hand, Keeping the thumb, ring finger and little finger extended.
- Close your right nostril with your thumb, and place the ring finger between your eyebrows. Inhale through the left nostril to a count of 5.

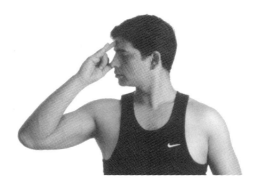

- Close the left nostril with the ring finger. Now both nostrils are closed. Hold your breath for a count of 10.

- Raise your thumb to the mid-point between your eyebrows and exhale slowly through the right nostril to a count of 10.
- Breathe in again through the right nostril to a count of 5.
- Close the right nostril with your thumb. Both the nostrils are closed now. Hold your breath for 10.
- Move the ring finger to the mid-point between your eyebrows and exhale through the left nostril to a count of 10.
- This completes one cycle of the *pranayama*. Repeat the complete cycle for two to five minutes.

Note

The ratio of *purak* (inhalation): *kumbhak* (holding breath): *rechak* (exhalation) is 1:2:2 in the beginning and can finally be 1:4:2, which is the ideal ratio.

Benefits

- Improves concentration and other mental faculties.
- Provides mental relaxation, particularly to people engaged in mental work.

Contraindication

- People with high blood pressure should not hold their breath for long.

MAHABANDHA

- Sit in *padmasana* preferably, or *sukhasana* with your eyes closed. You can also sit on a chair with you back straight, and legs kept apart, if sitting on the floor is difficult.
- Exhale forcefully through the mouth, and retain the breath outside.
- Lock your chin against your chest (*jalandhar bandha*).
- Suck in your stomach to create a hollow space (*udyaan bandha*).
- Squeeze and contract your anal area and pull upwards. Your lower abdominal muscles should be tightly contracted (*mool bandha*), as long as comfortable.
- Release in sequence — first the anal muscles, followed by the stomach muscles, and finally the chin lock.
- Look up and inhale. Repeat three times.

Benefits

- Gives benefits of all three *bandhas*.
- Checks the ageing process and keeps the mind cool.

Caution

- Do not attempt the *mahabandha* until all the three other *bandhas* have been mastered.

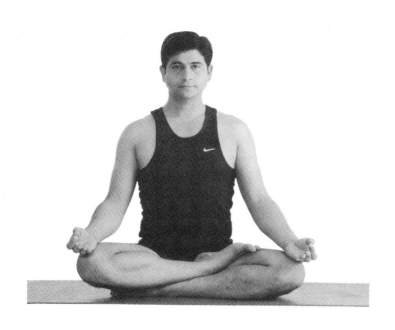

ARDHA MATSYENDRASANA (half spinal twist)

- Sit straight with your legs stretched out. Bend the left knee, placing it under the right leg, with the foot close to the right buttock.
- Bend the right knee, and place the right leg across the left knee.
- With your left hand, lock the right knee in place. This is done by holding on to the right foot; else, place the left hand on the left knee or simply hold the right knee with your left palm or elbow.
- Place the free hand behind the back.
- Twist the back as much as possible and look backwards.
- Hold this position for 10 to 30 seconds, and breathe normally.

Benefits

- This *asana* is ideal for management of diabetes as it exerts pressure on the pancreas, aiding in secretion of insulin.
- Stretches the back, increasing its flexibility, toning the spinal nerves and relieving muscular spasms.
- Massages abdominal organs and alleviates digestive ailments.

Contraindications

- Pregnant women suffering from hernia, hyperthyroidism and peptic ulcer should avoid this posture.

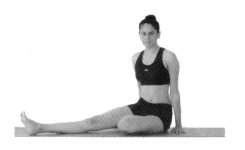
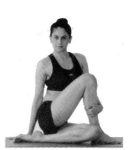
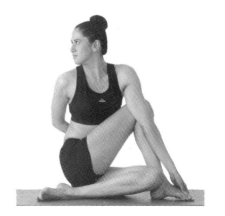

GOMUKHASANA

- Sit with your back straight and legs stretched out.
- Bend the left knee, and place the foot beside the right buttock.
- Now bend the right knee and place it over the left knee, with the foot beside the left buttock or sit in a simple crossed-legged position, keeping the back straight.
- Raise your left hand above the head. Bend it and place it behind your shoulders, palm on the back.
- Bend your right hand and take it backwards from under the armpit, reach out for the left hand, and interlock your fingers.
- Pull the arms gently away from each other, with your back straight. Remain thus for 10 to 30 seconds, breathing normally.
- Repeat the procedure on the other side.

Benefits

- Increases flexibility of the arms and shoulder blades.
- Clears the chest, helps in respiration and tones the back.

Contraindication

- Persons with frozen shoulder should avoid this *asana*.

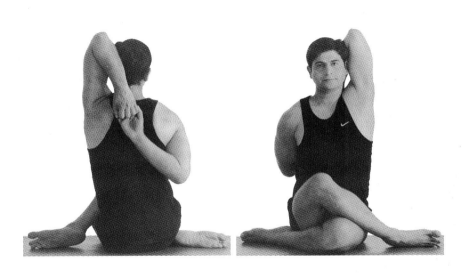

113

TIRYAKA BHUJANGASANA

- Do *bhujangasana*.
- Slowly exhaling, turn your back and head and look over your left shoulder.
- Try to look at your right heel.
- Breathe normally.
- Hold this posture for a few seconds.
- Return to *bhujangasana* and to the floor.
- Repeat the entire practice and turn the body to the other side.
- *Tiryaka bhujangasana* should be practiced only once the back is sufficiently flexible and strong.

Benefits

- Stretches the sides of the abdominal area, exerting a mild pressure on the internal organs including the pancreas.
- Stretches and strengthens the back and the neck muscles.

Contraindications

- People with severe backache should avoid this *asana*.
- Persons who have recently undergone surgery in the abdominal area should consult their doctor before attempting this *asana*.

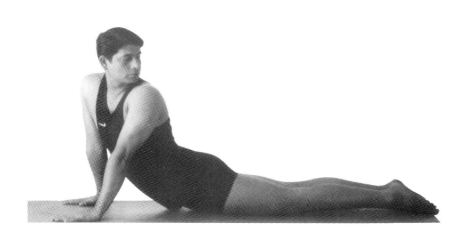

DHANURASANA (bow pose)

- Lie on your stomach.
- Fold your knees and reach behind to hold your ankles.
- Inhale and raise the body up.
- Arch your body backwards while pushing upwards with your legs. Try to keep the chest and thighs off the ground, with only the abdominal area touching the ground.
- Breathe normally and hold the position for 10 to 30 seconds.

Benefits

- Stretches the abdominal area, exerting a mild pressure on the pancreas.
- Strengthens the back and removes mild backache.
- Stretches and massages the abdominal muscles, removing excess fat from this area.

Contraindication

- People with severe lumbar and cervical pain should avoid this *asana*.

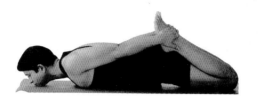

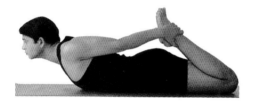

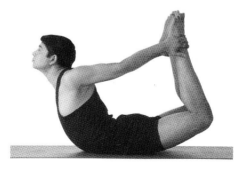

NAUKASANA (boat pose)

- Lie flat on your back, arms by the sides.
- Inhale and raise your legs 45 degrees above the ground.
- Raise the upper body 45 degrees above the ground.
- Stretch your arms straight out beside your thighs, so that the body makes a 'boat' shape.
- Breathe normally and hold the posture for 10 to 30 seconds. If holding is difficult, initially practice three times with the hold periods lasting 10 seconds each.

Benefits

- Exerts a mild pressure on the pancreas.
- Strengthens and tones the abdomen muscles, taking the excess weight off your abdominal area.
- Strengthens the back and thigh muscles.

Contraindications

- Those with neck problems should avoid this *asana*.
- Persons with lower back problems should also avoid this *asana*.

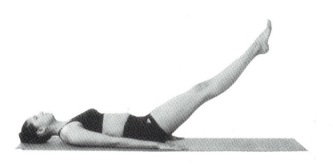

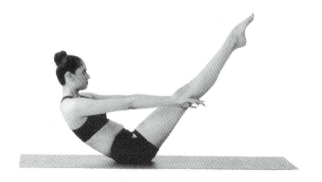

VIPREETKARNIASANA

- Lie on your back with your hands by your sides.
- Slowly raise both your legs.
- Bring them to a 90-degree position.
- Lift your hips and support them with your hands.
- Breathe normally and hold for 10 to 30 seconds.

Benefits

- Clears blockages in the arteries of the heart.
- Improves blood circulation in the face and the upper parts of the body.
- Helps in removing pimples, patches on the face and pigmentation while improving the glow on the face.
- Assists in healthy hair growth, stops premature greying of hair and hair fall to a great extent.

Contraindication

- People suffering from hernia, high blood pressure or spinal injury should avoid practicing this *asana*.

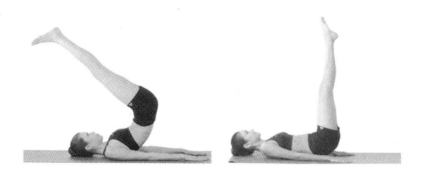

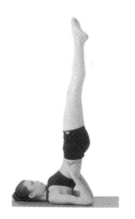

MATSYAASANA

- This *asana* is contrary to the chin lock of *vipreetkarniasana*.
- Sit in *padmasana*, or sit with your legs stretched out.
- Lie down on your back with palms under your buttocks and elbows on the floor.
- Raise your upper body, supporting yourself on your elbows.
- Push your chest outwards and drop your head backwards, resting the crown of your head on the floor.
- Place your hands on the thighs and relax in this posture.
- Hold this position for 10 to 30 seconds. To return, raise your head and upper body, supporting yourself on your elbows.
- Slowly lower your back to the floor and remove hands from under the buttocks.

Benefits

- Breaks the lock produced by *sarvangasana*, besides removing a double chin and cervical spondylosis.
- Strengthens the neck and shoulder muscles.

Contraindications

- People suffering from severe cervical problems should consult an orthopaedic surgeon before doing this *asana*.
- If you suffer from a spinal injury, avoid this *asana*.

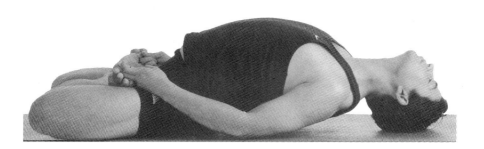

MEDITATION

Continue with your practice of *ajapa japa* by increasing the time. You can practice *yognidra* immediately after the practice of *ajapa japa*. *Yognidra* is a very important for inducing relaxation and can also be practiced if you have difficulty in sleeping.

YOGNIDRA

Yognidra is an ancient art of yogic meditation that helps one to enter the deepest part of consciousness.

- Lie down on your back on a hard mattress.
- Cover yourself with a white clean sheet up to your neck, wearing the minimum of clothes.
- Play soothing music (instrumental) in the background.
- Become aware of your breath.
- Inhale and exhale a few times.
- Allow the breath to become deeper and breathe from your abdomen approximately for two to five minutes.

There are 16 vital points in the human body, which can totally relax you if your become aware of them. These points are the toes, ankles, calves, knees, thighs, abdomen, chest, shoulders, elbows, wrist, fingertips, neck, chin, lips, nostrils and the forehead. Move from the forehead to your toes and vice-versa two to three times.

- Imagine that your limbs are detached from your main body and that only your head, chest and abdominal area exist.

- Breathe and feel the air enter your spine, cleaning the whole spinal column via the *prana*.
- Become aware of the different vital *chakras* (plexus group of nerves) present in your body by starting from the *mooladhara* (root plexus, the point between the anal space and the genital), move to the *swadhisthan* (the point which is four fingers below the navel region), then *manipurak* (the point four fingers above the navel region), *anahath* (the mid point of the chest), *vishuddhi* (mid point of the throat), *aghya* (point between the eyebrows), and lastly, *sahasraar* (mid point of the skull).

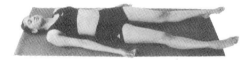

- Breathe in and out at every *chakra*, five to 10 times.
- Feel your limbs getting attached to the body. Be aware of your whole body for some time as one unit.
- Slowly open your eyes and get up. An important point to be remembered while practicing *yognidra* is that one should avoid sleeping.